CONVERSATIONS THAT MATTER

guy·ology ®

JUST THE FACTS

A Guy's Guide to Growing Up

MELISA HOLMES, MD
TRISH HUTCHISON, MD
with help from our favorite guys

3LEAF Press
Charleston, South Carolina

Illustrations by Lisa Perrett
Cover Design by Ashley Inzer

Table of Contents

We talk with parents of boys and girls ages 8 to 18 on a daily basis. If you are like most of them, we know that you want the best for your children. We know that you want them to have better information than you did about growing up. We also know that you lack a little confidence when it comes to talking with them about puberty, reproduction, and their emerging sexuality. We started Girlology and Guyology to help. We're here to give you some information, some tips, and some gentle nudging to start talking—*now*.

It's true that puberty is beginning at younger and younger ages for both girls and boys. And although their bodies are changing, they may lack the emotional and cognitive abilities that help them navigate their emerging sexuality. They need your help.

Now, more than ever, children need you to provide honest and accurate sexuality education. Research confirms that children want to hear it from you more than from their school, the media, or even their friends. But if your kids get the idea that you may be bluffing or hiding some of the truth, they'll turn to their ultimate authority: the Internet. And that should really make you panic.

This book is a great starting place for boys who are facing or just entering puberty. We present everything about puberty, and nothing about intercourse. That makes it easier for them to process without getting overwhelmed with too much information.

When boys and girls learn about what to expect *before* it happens, they face puberty with greater confidence and even a little excitement.

We encourage you to read this book, too, so you know what information your son has.

Most of all, do your best to be open and honest when he asks questions or wants to talk about something—no matter how awkward it may be. Establishing yourself as his go-to person for sexuality education creates an important parent–child connection that will protect him for years to come.

Good luck!

Melisa Holmes, MD, and Trish Hutchison, MD
Co-founders, Girlology and Guyology

CHAPTER 1

Here's the Deal

Growing up? Really? Did a parent just give you this book? Did you roll your eyes, or were you a little excited? Either would be normal because this book is going to give you a lot of information that may seem awkward, but it's really important. It's about puberty—that time when your body starts changing to look more grown up.

Now that you're getting older, you need to understand what to expect when puberty starts. You need to know how your body will change and how to take care of it. And honestly, it's pretty interesting.

The most important thing to understand as you head toward puberty is that **you will have the same body changes that all guys have but they will happen on your own unique timeline, and you will end up with your own unique look when it's over.**

That means puberty can be confusing or frustrating because it's a bit of a mystery. When will your changes start? When will they finish? What will you look like when it's all done?

The title of this book is *Guyology: Just the Facts*, because we're going to stick to just the facts of puberty. You may already know that talking about puberty can lead to other awkward conversations, but we are going to stick to puberty for now.

So, what exactly does puberty mean?

It's a strange-sounding word, but it comes from two Latin words: *Pubertas* means to become more adult-like. That seems about right.

And then there's *pubescere*, which means "to become ripe" or "to grow hairy or mossy."

Hmmm. There is definitely some hairiness that will happen, so maybe that's pretty accurate, too.

Putting it simply, **puberty is a time when your body begins to grow up and become more adultlike.**

Why?

Your body has to go through these changes so that one day you can mate and repopulate the human species. In other words, help make a baby. That means that your "private parts" are getting an extreme makeover and your body is changing from a boy's body to a man's body.

Everyone goes through puberty, but not everyone gets the chance to learn how and why it happens. Learning about this stuff might make you feel excited, interested, embarrassed, or just plain awkward. That's normal. Keep reading, and you'll see that it will get easier and more interesting.

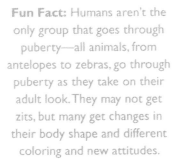

Fun Fact: Humans aren't the only group that goes through puberty—all animals, from antelopes to zebras, go through puberty as they take on their adult look. They may not get zits, but many get changes in their body shape and different coloring and new attitudes.

Girls

Obviously, this book is all about Guyology, but you also need to understand a little about girls' puberty, too. Understanding the changes that happen to girls and boys makes you smarter, and it's important to know. Yep. Gotta do it.

Do girls go through puberty? Of course. Boys and girls both have to grow up and have body changes. Some of the changes are the same for boys and girls (like growing taller), but a lot of the changes are different since boys' and girls' bodies are different (we bet you knew that). We'll talk mostly about boys' changes in this book, but we just want to make sure you understand girls' changes, too.

Let's start by comparing the changes that girls and boys will go through. Look at the list below and decide whether it's a puberty change that happens to girls, boys, or both. You can draw a line from each change to the girl or boy picture. You may not even know what some of these things mean. That's OK. You'll know about everything on this list if you keep reading. The answers are at the end of the chapter.

Who Does What?

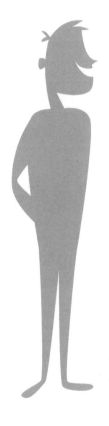

sweat more

hairy legs

feelings change

shoulders get wider

pimples

facial hair

body odor

testicles grow

grow taller

pubic hair

breasts grow

erections happen more

underarm hair

periods begin

voice changes

oily skin and hair

penis grows

chest hair

hips get wider

bigger muscles

ejaculations begin

Adam's apple grows

Did you realize that boys have more changes happening than girls do? It's fun to have a friendly competition with girls sometimes, but don't try that when it comes to puberty because, even though guys have a longer list of changes, girls almost always start developing before boys do.

For girls, puberty can start as young as age 7 or as late as age 12. We'll talk more about their changes in Chapter 10.

Boys don't usually start puberty until a little later, which can be as early as age 8 or as late as age 14. It might be nice to get it all over with quickly, but puberty will last around 5 years. **It takes a long time to make a masterpiece,** and that's sort of what's happening.

If you see middle school kids, you may have noticed that the girls are taller than a lot of the boys. That's because girls grow faster around ages 11 to 12, and boys grow faster around age 13 or 14. So, even though girls get a head start and are taller than the boys in early middle school, most boys end up taller because their growth spurt lasts longer.

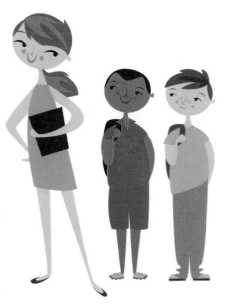

So, boys have a LOT of changes, and you probably have a lot of questions: Why does it start? What exactly will happen? How do I handle it? Why do I feel so weird sometimes? We'll try to answer all of these questions, but let's start by making sure you know the details about stuff "down there" because, for boys, that's where it all begins.

Here are the answers for you.

BOYS	GIRLS
sweat more	sweat more
hairy legs	hairy legs
feelings change	feelings change
shoulders get wider	hips get wider
pimples	pimples
facial hair	facial hair
body odor	body odor
testicles grow	grow taller
grow taller	pubic hair
pubic hair	breasts grow
breasts grow	periods begin
erections happen more	underarm hair
underarm hair	oily skin and hair
voice changes	
oily skin and hair	
penis grows	
chest hair	
bigger muscles	
ejaculations begin	
Adam's apple grows	

CHAPTER 2

AWKwords

GO!

EAT
MORE!

LET OUT
THE STINK!

READY TO
GROW!

GROW, GROW, GROW!

Have you ever heard your mom or dad mention **hormones?** Sometimes, hormones are blamed for bad things—like cranky moods or crazy behavior—but hormones are actually good things. They act as chemical messengers that help our body parts communicate with each other. Hormones help us fall asleep, they tell our bodies when to grow, they control our energy, and they tell us when to feel hungry and how much pee to make. Guess what else they control? Yep. Puberty.

So, puberty begins as your brain sends out hormones to tell your body to grow and change. **The actual moment when your brain says go is sort of a mystery.** Scientists still haven't figured out exactly what makes it happen when it does, but it happens for everyone at some point!

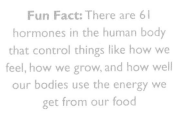

What's Happening?

Growing is one of the first signs of puberty. There's a hormone called growth hormone (that's easy) that increases a bunch during puberty. But it's not like you are a kid when you go to sleep and a full-grown man when you wake up. This growth hormone affects your body size over a long time, and it starts somewhere you might not expect. Actually, before all the "private stuff" starts happening, your hands and feet start to grow!

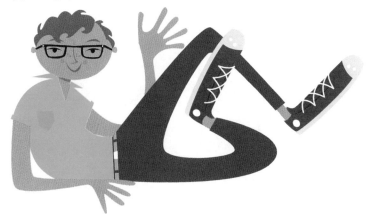

Have you noticed you are growing out of your shoes more rapidly? That could be the signal that puberty is starting. Have you also noticed that your feet stink more when they are growing fast? True. But that's a different topic. We'll talk more about odors in Chapter 7.

You probably already know that the fun doesn't end there. There's another hormone called testosterone that causes most of the puberty changes for boys. A tiny, pea-sized gland in the brain, called the pituitary gland, sends a chemical messenger (yep, another hormone) to the testicles (or maybe you know them as your "balls") to tell them to start making testosterone.

Silly Willy

Speaking of balls, we all hear silly names for our private body parts. You know some, don't you? Go ahead, write down some of your special names for your private parts:

Did you mention weiner? dick? balls? nuts? willy? junk? ding dong? one-eyed snake?

Why do we have such silly names for our body parts? Sure, talking about this stuff can be pretty embarrassing. Those parts are private, right? And being private means that you keep them to yourself and nobody else can look at them or touch them (unless it's your doctor and he or she has your permission and your parents' permission). And nobody should ask you to look at or touch their private parts or anybody else's. Private, right?

Privacy Matters

Why is the privacy thing so important? Sometimes there are people (very wrong people) who want to look at or touch children's private parts or have children look at or touch theirs. Sometimes these people are older kids. Sometimes they are even family members or someone you know and trust. They think they can talk children into keeping this a secret, or pretend it's a game, or scare kids into thinking they've done something bad. They try to make children keep it a secret.

The truth is, this is called sexual abuse, and adults who do it are called **pedophiles** or **sexual abusers**. Sexual abuse happens more than you might think even though it is very, very wrong and against the law. If anyone ever tries to involve you in something like this, it's really important to tell an adult you trust. If it has happened to you, it's not your fault, and you won't get in trouble for it. Telling an adult can make it stop and keep the abuser from doing that to other children, too. Don't ever keep it a secret.

Down There Parts

So, there are lots of silly names out there, but it's also important that you know the correct names for your body parts. If you ever get hurt or have a problem with your body, particularly your private areas, it's important for you to be able to tell a doctor or your parents what's wrong. You'll need the right names to do that.

This is where you have a distinct advantage over girls: knowing your parts.

Girls' parts are kind of hidden around a corner and between some folds. Yours are just hanging right there in front of you. All you have to do is look down, and there they are.

Since you were a baby, you've been looking at and touching your parts, right? And when you were potty trained, you had to hold your penis to aim it into the toilet. So if you're like most boys, you have been pretty familiar with your outside private parts for a long time.

You probably know the names, too, but let's go through them just to be sure:

Penis: This is the part that hangs down in front of your body that you pee (urinate) from. It is made up of two parts: the head (also called the glans) and the shaft.

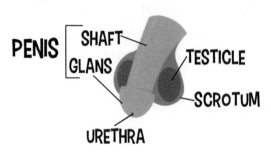

PENIS ⌈ SHAFT
      ⌊ GLANS   TESTICLE
                 SCROTUM
URETHRA

Testicle: You have two of them, and they hang in a sack of skin behind your penis. You may know them as your balls or nuts. Your testicles are where testosterone comes from, and they are really important in the repopulating mission. The plural form of the word "testicle" is "testes," although a lot of people say testicles. We know what you're talking about whether you use testicles or testes, but just so you sound really smart, the proper word for two balls is testes. So there.

Gonad: Another word for testicle.

Scrotum: This is the sack of skin that holds the testes. This little sack may seem simple, but it actually has some pretty special powers as a thermoregulator (that means it helps control the temperature of your testes). Why would it need to do that? Don't worry, we'll answer that eventually. Keep reading.

Urethra: This is the hole at the tip of your penis that your pee, or urine, comes out of (you probably call it your pee hole).

Anus: Your anus is the hole that your poop comes out of. (You probably call it your butt hole. Now you know better.) You may notice that some kids giggle when your science teacher talks about the solar system and mentions the planet Uranus, as in "Uranus is a

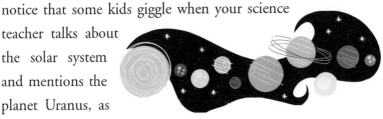

gassy planet." Your science teacher may even giggle. Something about that just makes us laugh sometimes. It's OK. We just want to make sure you know the correct words for all of your parts, including this one!

Circumcision

All boys are born with a piece of skin, called the foreskin, covering the head (glans) of the penis. Some parents choose to have the foreskin removed, and that is called circumcision. When a boy is circumcised, the foreskin is removed by a doctor (or rabbi or mohel in the Jewish faith). Some parents choose to have this done for religious reasons soon after a boy is born or just so their son's penis looks like Dad's (if Dad is circumcised). Some parents choose to leave the foreskin as it is. Sometimes a boy can't be circumcised right after birth because of a health reason, so he may be circumcised later or not at all. Even though most circumcisions are done on babies, a boy or man can be circumcised at any age.

Fun Fact: Scientists have discovered how to use the foreskins from circumcised babies to grow new skin in the laboratory. In just a few weeks, a single foreskin can grow enough new skin to cover three basketball courts! This laboratory-grown skin can be used to treat patients with bad burns

It is normal if you are circumcised, and it's also normal if you are not. Even though a circumcised penis looks a bit different than an uncircumcised one, they work just the same.

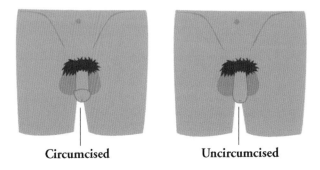

Circumcised   **Uncircumcised**

If you are not circumcised, you will have to pay a little more attention to cleaning your penis. It is important for you to pull back the foreskin when you take a bath or shower so that you can clean under the foreskin. If soap stings it, then just use water. If you can't pull your foreskin back very far, that's OK. Over time it will loosen up, and you will be able to pull it all the way back when you get older. Don't ever force the foreskin back if it hurts. If it ever feels tight or becomes red or swollen, you'll need to tell your parents and see your doctor.

So, as a young boy, your outside private parts are pretty simple. But you're not so young anymore. As puberty begins, things will start to change down there and on other parts of your body, too. In the next chapter, we'll go over how the changes start and what to expect.

CHAPTER 3

It's Starting for Real

Now that you know the correct names for your parts, let's talk about the changes that are about to happen to them. It's always nice to know what's next, right? You already know that your feet and hands will grow quickly as puberty begins. But bigger hands and feet don't seem like such a big deal. You'll know it's the real deal of puberty when your private parts start changing.

Nobody Wants a Puberty Surprise

Remember, the good news is that the changes happen slowly. That means, you won't wake up one morning with a man-size penis and a body covered in hair. That would be freaky. Instead, **these changes happen gradually over 4 to 5 years.** So it's not a sprint but more of an endurance race.

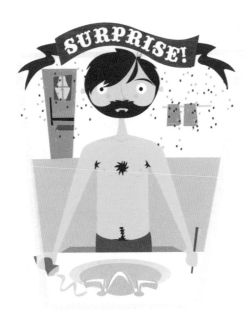

Believe it or not, there was a doctor a long time ago that decided to organize all the body changes that happen during puberty into steps or stages. His name was Dr. Tanner, and the stages of growth were named Tanner Stages. Some doctors call these stages the Sexual Maturity Rating instead of Tanner Stages. We'll just call them puberty stages.

Now why do we need to describe each stage of puberty? Well, it helps you and your doctor know that your body parts are growing and changing like they should. Plus, it helps you to know what to expect. Nobody wants a puberty surprise.

The first two stages of puberty are described below. You can read through them to see where you are and figure out what's next.

Puberty Stage 1 (Prepuberty)

Dr. Tanner didn't make a Stage Zero, so Stage 1 is where everyone starts as little kids. Stage 1 is what your body looks like before puberty truly starts. It means there have been no changes yet. So that means . . .

* Your penis and testes are the same size that they've been most of your life.

* You don't have any hair down there—just maybe a little "peach fuzz."

* You are growing taller at the same speed you have been growing since you were a toddler. That's about 2 inches (5 to 6 cm) per year.

* Your hands and feet will grow faster at the end of Stage 1, but you may not even notice when that happens!

Puberty Stage 2 (The True Beginning)

Stage 2 is the actual starting line for the real deal of puberty. It can start anytime between ages 8 and 14, but the average age is around 9 to 11. As a boy, **the real deal of puberty begins between**

your legs, so you may not even notice exactly when it starts. Here's what happens:

* Your testes will grow first.
* Your scrotum will stretch with your growing testes and will become a darker color.
* You will have darker hairs begin to sprout at the base of your penis. They are straight at first and become curly over time.
* You may or may not have dark hairs growing in your armpits.
* Your penis begins to grow longer.
* You may notice changes in the color and size of your nipples. They may also be a little sore or tender.
* Your hands and feet seem too large for the rest of your body because they are growing fast, but you are not getting a lot taller.
* You will begin to have erections more often and at unpredictable times.

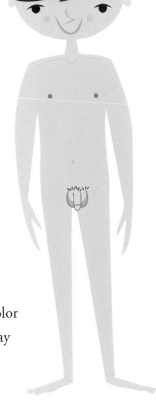

Fun Fact: If you have a few hairs (enough that you can count them all), you are definitely in Stage 2. If you have more hairs than you can easily count, you have probably progressed to Stage 3. Congratulations!

Wait. What?

Erection Section

Erections? Let's talk about those for a minute, just so you have the facts.

The word "erect" means "tall and straight," and that's exactly what happens to your penis with an erection. So, an erection is when your penis gets hard and sticks up. You've been having erections all your life, but you may not have paid much attention to them. Even baby boys have erections—sometimes when they have to pee or when they play with their penis.

Do you know why or how it happens? Well, some people call it a "boner," but we promise, you don't grow a bone in there.

The penis is made of two tubes that are filled with spongelike stuff. Each tube also has a blood vessel running through the middle of it. An erection happens when the blood fills the spongy area so tightly that it makes the penis stiff and erect. But don't worry—you won't see that blood. It just fills in the space, then goes back to where it came from. It won't come out of your penis or anything scary like that.

Once you have started puberty, you will get erections that may happen when you least expect it. It's sort of like blushing.

Sometimes you know what will make you blush, and sometimes you have no idea! It can be pretty random.

When it comes to erections, it's sort of like that. Most guys think they occur only when they are thinking about girls or something "sexy." But there are lots of other things that might trigger an erection. Sometimes it might happen just because you see something that excites you, like a shiny, fast new car. You can also have one if you are sitting on something that is vibrating or tickling your privates, like a running car or even the school bus. **And sometimes, erections just happen for no reason at all, and they can happen a lot!** For a lot of guys, waking up with an erection is an everyday thing. And honestly, during puberty, erections are really, really common, and you don't have a lot of control over when they do or don't happen.

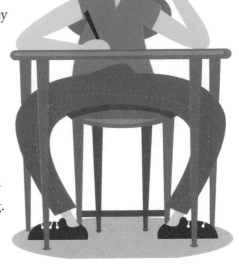

When you have a surprise erection (and you will), it can feel really embarrassing. First, you need to know that other people probably can't see it and have no idea it's happening. But, if you're worried that others can see it, then

there are some things you can do to
keep it hidden until it's gone away.

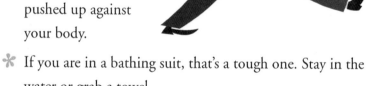

* If you are sitting, don't
  stand up.

* If you have to stand up, you
  can untuck your shirt or
  carry a book or backpack in
  front of you to cover yourself.

* You can put your hand
  in your pocket to hold
  it down or keep it
  pushed up against
  your body.

* If you are in a bathing suit, that's a tough one. Stay in the
  water or grab a towel.

* Get to a private place, like a restroom.

Here are some other tips on controlling them:

* Briefs will keep them hidden better than boxers will.

* Taking your mind off of it can help it go away, so
  sometimes you can try thinking about something boring
  or focusing on something like multiplication tables.

As you get older and progress through puberty, you won't have
as many random erections. But in the early and middle stages of
puberty, it's good to know what to expect and how to manage them.

Protecting Your Parts

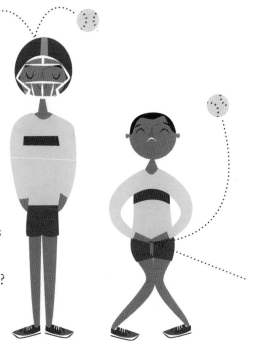

Now that these parts are getting bigger, there are a few things you need to know so you can protect them, because one day, they'll have an important mission to accomplish (repopulating is pretty important).

Do you play any sports? Sports can be a great way to make friends and get exercise, but injuries happen. Have you ever been hit in the testes (balls)? If you have, you'll understand why protecting your privates is helpful.

Some of your body parts have built-in protection. Your rib cage protects your heart and lungs, your skull protects your brain, and muscles protect your stomach, but your penis and testes are left hanging with nothing. Because of their "loose" location outside the body, they can get hit, knocked, and kicked pretty easily. They can survive most hits without being permanently injured because they are spongy. But, if your testes are bumped, it definitely hurts, like nothing you've ever felt before. Most guys describe it as a horrible feeling that they feel more in their gut, like getting kicked in the stomach by a horse. If your testes are hit hard, you might even feel like throwing up. The pain should go away within an hour. If it doesn't, you may need to see your doctor.

If you are hit hard in the testes or penis, here are some things you can do to make it feel better:

* Stop playing.

* Lie down.

* Bend your knees or pull them up toward your belly.

* Place an ice pack over your testes.

* If it's OK with your parents, you may want to take a pain reliever, such as ibuprofen.

You should call your doctor if any of the following things happen:

* The pain gets worse or lasts more than an hour.

* You notice bruising or swelling.

* You have a hard time urinating (peeing).

* Your urine (pee) looks pink or bloody.

Straps and Compression

If you are involved in team sports, your coach may tell you to get compression shorts or an athletic cup. **This type of protection is just as important as your helmet and mouth guard.** In fact, men decided a long time ago that it was important to protect their privates.

The first jockstrap was invented in 1874 to provide comfort and support for men riding bicycles on the cobblestone streets of Boston. The first athletic cup was invented and used the same year in the sport of ice hockey. Know what's sort of odd? The first helmet (for protecting your brain!) was not used in sports until 20 years later! Do you think they valued their man-parts more than their brains?!

Just to make sure you know the details, a jockstrap is a type of athletic support made of stretchy, snug fabric that holds your penis and testes securely in place. Today, most guys use compression shorts instead. These are soft shorts that are tight but stretchy. They kind of squeeze everything in close to your body.

It's challenging to run hard if your private parts are swinging and slapping around uncomfortably. Compression shorts keep that from happening. It is really important to make sure you have the right size. If your compression shorts aren't snug, they won't do their job.

Cups

The other way to protect yourself is with an athletic cup. It's basically a piece of hard plastic that protects your penis and testes from injury. If you've ever been hit or kicked in the testes, you'll know why it's important. If you haven't, trust us. Protecting your "parts" can save you a lot of pain. There's no need to use an athletic cup when you're just hanging around or running, but **if you are participating in a contact sport or a sport involving a ball, puck, or other flying object, an athletic cup is important.** In fact, these sports leagues usually require you to wear one:

* Football
* Baseball
* Hockey
* Lacrosse

Putting It On

To wear an athletic cup, you will need compression shorts. You can't just wear the cup inside your boxers, and you don't want the cup directly against your skin. Compression shorts have a pocket or pouch that the cup can slide into.

It seems strange at first because you have to make sure your penis and testes are placed correctly. Point the cup so that the skinny end points downward between your legs, then insert it in the pouch in the compression shorts. As you pull on the shorts,

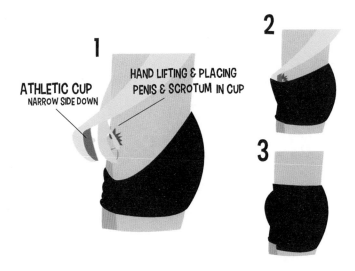

1 — ATHLETIC CUP NARROW SIDE DOWN — HAND LIFTING & PLACING PENIS & SCROTUM IN CUP

2

3

lift your penis and testes up, then place them comfortably inside the cup as you press the cup against your body. Your compression shorts will hold the cup in the correct position. Once you get used to it, it should become as routine as putting on your helmet or other safety gear.

CHAPTER 4

A Busy Body

What's challenging for a lot of boys is that nobody notices they have started puberty until they start growing taller, have voice cracks, or grow hairier. That's because there is a lot of stuff that happens "down there" before anyone sees the other changes and even thinks about their needing privacy.

What a Man!

By the time you get to Tanner Stage 3, it will start to become obvious to everyone that puberty is well under way. You'll hear comments like "Wow! You are growing up!" or "Look at you! You're turning into a young man." As awkward as these comments may be, you'll finally start to get your well-deserved privacy and understanding. But until folks can see the changes, **you may need to remind them that there are things "going on" down there and you would appreciate some privacy.**

Puberty Stage 3 (Growing)

Once you have finished Stage 2 and are heading into Stage 3, things really start to take off, especially your height. Stage 3 can start anytime between ages 10 and 16, but on average, it happens around ages 12 to 13, which is usually toward the middle or end of middle school. By this time, you are growing about 3 inches each year, and you're not even growing at full speed yet! You've never grown this fast, and that's why it can hurt sometimes. Yes, growing pains are real.

GROWTH CHART
4 MONTHS!!
4 YEARS

But growing taller is only one of many things happening in this stage. There are more changes happening "down there." There are also changes happening with your hair, your body, your appetite, and even your moods. Let's break it all down.

Below the Belt

Once you get to Stage 3, things will start to look a lot different below your belt. Your penis grows longer, and the glans (head) of your penis may get darker in color. Along with that, your testes continue to grow, and the scrotum allows one testicle to hang lower than the other. That's a nice way to keep them from bumping together. It might be interesting to know that it is more common for the left testicle to hang lower than the right one. But, **just like being**

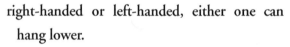

right-handed or left-handed, either one can hang lower.

The scrotum also takes on another job as thermoregulator to keep your testes happy. That means that when you're hot, your scrotum drops lower to stay cool. And when you're cold, it pulls in closer to your body to keep your testes cozy and warm. This seems pretty cool and a little strange, but it's actually important for the way your body works. More on that later.

Hair Ninja

Remember the word for puberty that means "to grow hairy or mossy"? This is when you'll start to see the true meaning of growing hairier. It's like the hair ninja pays you a visit and makes you sprout hair in the most awkward places! Your hair around your penis (called pubic hair) becomes darker, curlier, and begins to spread. By this time, there are definitely more hairs than you would want to count. The hair in your armpits will also begin to fill in more. By then, you will have noticed that your

Fun Fact: Your scalp has about 615 hair follicles per square centimeter. The thickness and color of your hairs are inherited from your ancestors. So is baldness. On average, most adults have about 5 million hair follicles over their entire body, and that number never changes, but hairs may fall out of follicles and never grow back

leg and arm hair is darker and thicker, too. You can thank the hair ninja.

Noticing Nipples

You probably know that girls grow breasts in puberty. But did you know that some boys do, too? Yes, boys have breasts, too. They just don't grow or have the same function as girls' breasts (for feeding babies someday).

As you go through puberty, you may notice that your nipples and the surrounding dark ring, called the areola, get larger and darker. Also one or both of your breasts may start to stick up or even hurt a little. If your breasts grow, it's called gynecomastia (guy nuh coh MAST eeya). This can be totally normal, and it does not mean you will have "moobs" (man boobs) for the rest of your life.

Don't freak out.

It's actually normal for lots of guys to have some breast growth during puberty. It almost always goes away on its own. If this happens to you, you can know that it's common and won't need any treatment to make it go away. But if you ever get worried about how your nipples (or any other body part) are growing, you can always talk to your doctor.

Cracking and Breaking

Some of your body changes are so obvious, but others sneak up on you and show up when you least expect it. Like voice changes.

As your body is growing, your voice box is growing, too (you just can't see it). On men, the voice box, also called the larynx (LAIR inks), is the boney lump in the middle of their neck. It's also called the Adam's apple. As the larynx grows, it causes your vocal cords to stretch, grow, and eventually become thicker. And as your vocal cords stretch, your voice will start to make funny sounds that people call cracks, breaks, or squeaks. Most boys just call it annoying.

The good news is that the **voice cracks last only a few months, and when your larynx is finished growing, you will have a new, deeper voice.** Think of your vocal cords like guitar strings. The thinner ones are higher, and the thicker ones make a lower, deeper sound. Your vocal cords are becoming thicker, and that makes your voice deeper.

The voice changes, like most other puberty changes in boys, are caused by testosterone. Testosterone is the hormone that comes mostly from your testicles. If you remove your testicles before puberty, your voice will never change.

It's interesting (but also pretty strange—no, very strange) that way back in the 1500s to 1800s, boys that sang in large, formal churches with beautiful, high voices were sometimes castrated (meaning their testes were removed). By doing that, their voices stayed high, and they could continue to sing for the church for many more years. Gee. Makes you want to sing out of tune, huh? Thankfully, nobody does that anymore!

CHAPTER 5

Speed Growing

There's no magic line or measurement that tells you that you have moved from Stage 3 to Stage 4. Guys usually reach this stage between the ages of 12 and 18, and the average age is 14 or 15. The changes that have been happening, keep happening, but you'll also notice some new stuff. One of the biggest changes is how fast you are growing.

Puberty Stage 4 (Bigger Faster)

Stage 4 brings on the fastest growth you'll ever have. You may actually grow about 4 inches in a year!

All that growing can make you look a little funny and feel a bit awkward and clumsy. Your arms and legs are the first to do the "speed growing," so by the end of this stage, you may look extra long and lean. This happens because your bones are actually growing faster than your muscles are, and your muscles don't show up very well. Some guys are frustrated by this because looking strong and muscular seems cool (but being funny, brainy, or musical can be even cooler sometimes). No matter how you want your cool factor to shine, once you pass through Stage 4, your body will look more muscular and less lanky.

Trippy

And the clumsy part? That's normal, too. **As your bones grow faster than your muscles, it's totally normal to go through a clumsy stage.** This new clumsy phase happens because your muscles are being pulled and stretched as your bones are growing so fast. They can't keep up with all that bone growth, so they don't work as well. You may trip or stumble over your own feet, lose your balance more

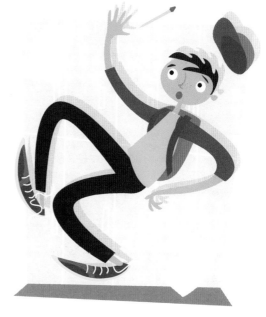

easily, or just not have the same moves that you've always had in sports or other activities. So be prepared to have some "off" times during your growth. It can be tough, but be patient and keep practicing. Once your muscles catch up with your bones and have a chance to adjust, you'll be even better than you were before you grew.

Ouch!

Growing pains may also continue through this stage. Normal growing pains feel like an ache inside your bones or muscles. If touching or squeezing an area makes it painful, that's probably not a growing pain but may be an injury instead. Also, if you are having normal growing pains, the pain will be in a general area, not just in one small spot that you can point to with the tip of your finger.

If growing pains keep you awake at night or interfere with your activities, you should check with your doctor. If your doctor examines you and finds nothing wrong, he or she may recommend a medicine for pain, like ibuprofen (Motrin, Advil) or naprosyn (Aleve). But always make sure you check with your parents before taking any medications. And if you are having pains that do not sound like normal growing pains, please see your doctor.

Down There

Yep, it's still changing down there. In this stage, your penis may grow a little longer, but it's also growing wider now. Your testicles and scrotum may hang even lower and become darker in color. This is also the stage that your body starts to make sperm. You may have heard of sperm, but let's make sure you know the facts.

Sperm

Remember that girls and boys all go through puberty so they can develop adult bodies that are able to repopulate the species (make babies) in the future. Making a new human is a pretty big deal. It takes a special cell from a male and a special cell from a female to make a new creature. Sperm is the name of the cell that comes from the male. And just to keep you sounding smart, one sperm is a sperm, and a million sperm are also called sperm (not sperms).

Your testes begin to make sperm once you reach this stage of puberty. And after that, your testes will continue to make sperm every day until you are an old man.

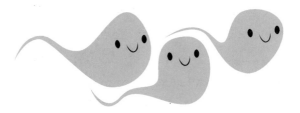

Sperm are tiny cells that look like tadpoles. Really, really tiny tadpoles. They have a rounded head and a longer section called a tail that allows them to swim. They are so small, you would never see a sperm

Fun Fact: Sperm can actually swim 3 millimeters per minute. Sounds slow, but when you're microscopic, that's pretty fast!

without a microscope. In fact, about 100 MILLION sperm can fit in a teaspoon.

Ejaculation

Once sperm are made in the testicles, they move into the epididymis (eh puh DID uh mus), where they spend a little time becoming mature (kind of like their own growing-up time). Eventually, the epididymis gets too crowded and the older, mature sperm have to go somewhere to make room for the newer "young" sperm. Sometimes, the older sperm will shrivel up and dissolve, but other times, they get out of your body by traveling through the vas deferens and out of your penis. When that happens, it's called ejaculation (ee JACK u lay shun). There's more about that in Chapter 6.

Fun Fact: A man's testes make about 10 million new sperm cells a day.

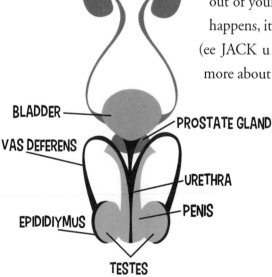

KIDNEYS

BLADDER

PROSTATE GLAND

VAS DEFERENS

URETHRA

PENIS

EPIDIDIYMUS

TESTES

So, along with this new sperm development, your body will begin to have ejaculations. Ejaculations happen only when your penis is erect, but just because you have an erection, doesn't mean you'll ejaculate. And even though you ejaculate through your penis, it's different than when you pee.

So, when does ejaculation happen? Sometimes, it can happen while you are sleeping. That's called a **nocturnal emission, or a wet dream**. It's totally nor-mal, but it can freak you out the first time it happens. If you are in Stage 4 of puberty and you wake up wet, it's probably a wet dream. How do you know you didn't pee in your bed? It will smell different than pee.

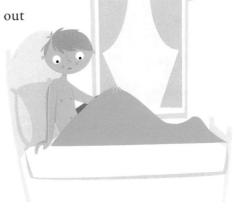

Make sure you figure out a plan with your parents. You can take the sheets off your bed and put them in the dirty laundry. Or you can learn how to wash and change your sheets by yourself. Don't just leave it there and think it will go away. If you leave it there, your sheets may feel stiff, and the smell may become pretty noticeable.

Masturbation

Ejaculation can also happen when you are touching your penis in a way that feels good. That's called masturbation (mas-ter BAY shun), but you may hear other silly words for it (like "playing with yourself," "jerking off," "jacking off," or "beating off"). Masturbation is something that guys tend to joke about or tease each other about. There are even some myths out there that you'll go blind or grow hair on your hands if you masturbate. All false! The truth is that masturbation feels good and most people think it's OK as long as you follow some basic rules:

* It's not a popular conversation for the dinner table.

* It's a private activity.

* It should not dominate your free time.

If you follow those simple rules, you should be fine. Masturbation is something that most people discover for themselves—and keep to themselves. But it's also something that most people do—some more than others.

Hair Ninja

Now, back to the other stuff, like the hair ninja. Yep, he's still at work in Stage 4, planting hairs on your face, sprouting more hair down there, and possibly sprinkling some on your chest (but not all guys get chest hair).

The hair on your face (facial hair) usually shows up first on your upper lip as a soft, wispy mustache. Then, it usually sprouts on your chin and near your ears as sideburns. The hairless spots will eventually fill in as you continue through puberty. For most guys, when the hair on their faces is noticeable or bothering them, they start shaving. When that time comes, you can look to Chapter 8 for some shaving tips.

And what happens to the "down there hair"? It may start to spread up to your navel and down onto your thighs. Some guys even get hair on their backs. **How hairy you become will depend on your ancestors and how hairy they were.**

Puberty Stage 5 (Manly)

Ta da! By this stage, you will be looking a lot more like a grown young man. It might be as early as age 14 or as late as in your 20s, but it's usually around ages 17 to 18. Even though your penis has finished growing, the hair ninja has done his job, and your muscles have filled in, your body shape can continue to change depending on how you treat it and feed it. It's important to take good care of this new body you're developing. We'll tell you how. Keep reading.

Penis Size

For whatever reasons, boys often worry about the size of their penises. Penises come in all different shapes and sizes. And the size of your penis is not at all related to the size of your other body parts despite what guys may say! Maybe some of you have heard that your penis size is related to your hand size, foot size, or even ear size! None of that is true.

Also, the size of your penis has nothing to do with how "manly" you are.

The average full-grown penis (when it is NOT erect) is 3 1/2 to 4 inches. With an erection, the average length is 5 to 6 inches. **And being larger or smaller than average doesn't mean your penis is any better or worse than anyone else's.**

Sometimes, your penis may even seem to bend to the left, to the right, or even up or down. It may look more bent than you think it should. This can be very normal. But if it worries you a lot or if the "bend" is ever painful during an erection, you should tell your doctor.

Just remember, we all come in different shapes and sizes (including penises), and that's a good thing.

CHAPTER 6

What's Going On in There?

So, we've talked a bunch about your outside, private guy parts. But what do you know about your inside parts? You probably know about some of them, so let's think about it. How do you know you have a heart? And what does it do? What about your lungs? And how do you know you have a liver?

um . . .

Well, you won't feel anything to tell you that your liver is in there, but trust us—it is. Your liver is in there and working because without it, you wouldn't be alive. So some of your inside parts may stay pretty quiet, but they are still very important.

Think about when you pee. That's a favorite activity isn't it? So now you know that your pee (urine) comes out of your urethra, but where does it come from before it comes out? Your

LUNGS

HEART

LIVER

BLADDER

TESTES

urine is stored in your bladder, which is on the inside. Sperm comes out of the urethra, too, but sperm doesn't come through the bladder. In fact, **you can't pee and ejaculate at the same time.** It's the inside parts that keep all that working just right.

So, obviously, **you have inside parts that are connected to your special outside parts.** Just to be complete, let's look at the inside parts that are connected up with your guy parts to see how they all work together.

Let's start with how urine comes out. Your kidneys make urine from the food and liquids you eat and drink. The kidneys send urine through some tubes into your bladder. Your bladder is like a storage unit for your urine. Once it gets full, the bladder tells your brain that you have to pee. Your brain will then allow the bladder valve to open into the urethra, which is actually a tube that passes through the penis, and allows your urine to exit at the tip. That's how your urine gets out.

Now, what about sperm? It has a longer journey.

As we mentioned in Chapter 5, it is made in the testes and stored in the **epididymis** (eh puh DID uh mus). When it's time to come out, it joins with some fluids from the **prostate gland** and **seminal vesicles**. The fluids make it easier for the sperm to swim (you can't swim without water, can you?), and they also provide nutrients (like snacks) for the journey. The sperm and the fluids together are called **semen** (SEA men). When ejaculation happens, the semen travels through tubes called the **vas deferens** into the penis and finally squirts out the tip of the penis through the urethra.

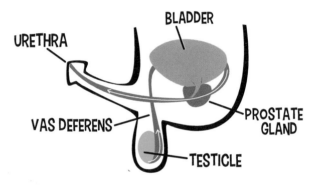

So urine and semen share the same exit, but they can't leave the body at the same time. In fact, there's a special valve that allows only one fluid to go through the urethra at a time. That helps keep the two fluids separated.

So how cool is that? **Your body is made in such an amazing way.** You can't pee and ejaculate at the same time, just like you can't breathe and swallow at the same time.

Here are a few more cool things to know about your guy-parts:

Testes: In humans, both of your testes are about the same size. In sharks, the right testicle is usually larger, and in many bird and mammal species, the left may be the larger. After puberty, the

Fun Fact: Human testicles are smaller than chimpanzee testicles but larger than gorilla testicles. That tells you bigger beasts don't always have bigger balls.

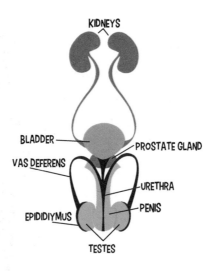

average testicle measures around 2 inches by 0.8 inch by 1.2 inches (or 5 x 2 x 3 cm).

Epididymis: Each testicle sends sperm into an epididymis, where the sperm are stored for up to 2 to 3 months. Each epididymis is actually a small but tightly coiled tube. If you stretched it out, it would be about 7 yards long! It's sort of an incubator where sperm mature and learn to swim.

Vas deferens: When ejaculation is about to occur, the sperm will leave each epididymis through two other tubes called the vas deferens on their way out to the penis. Each vas deferens is about 1 foot long. During ejaculation, these tubes help push the sperm forward. The sperm travels through the vas deferens into the urethra, collecting some of the fluids from the seminal vesicles and prostate gland along the way.

Prostate gland: The prostate gland is a little larger than a walnut, and it wraps around the urethra just below the bladder.

It adds fluid to the sperm to make up semen, and that fluid allows the sperm to swim better. You may have heard about prostate cancer in some older men (don't worry, it doesn't happen to young guys).

Urethra: This is the tube that connects the bladder and vas deferens to the end of the penis. It carries urine, as well as semen, but only one at a time. It is about 8 inches long in grown men.

Fun Fact: Do you think a big animal would have sperm bigger than a small animal's? The biggest sperm comes from a fruit fly! The sperm of a fruit fly can be as long as the body of the male fly, about 1.1 mm. Compared to other mammals, humans have one of the smallest sperm cells, measuring only 40 microns long (that's 0.004 mm, or four one-thousandths of a millimeter).

Bladder: Your bladder is the part of your body that holds or stores your urine before it needs to come out. The average bladder usually holds about 1 1/2 cups, or 300 to 350 ml of urine.

Kidneys: You have two kidneys, located in your midback area. They act like filters for your blood to pull out fluids, toxins, and waste to make urine. As the urine is made, it travels to the bladder through a tube called the ureter. Then it is stored in the bladder until it gets full and you have to pee.

So now you know your outside parts AND your inside parts. And you even know what they all do! Don't you feel smart?

CHAPTER 7

What's That Smell?

Just in case you don't have a nose to tell you, puberty can literally stink! If you walk into any middle school locker room, you'll probably notice a different smell hanging in the air. Some of that may be the perfume and body spray that middle schoolers like to pour on before school, but some of it (the stinky part) is the smell of puberty.

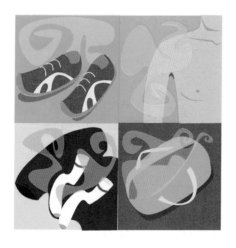

Sweat

What's the big deal about sweat? All your life, you've been sweating. But here's the deal. In puberty, you'll sweat more than ever. Sometimes

you'll sweat just because you are hot
or exercising, but in puberty, you
may also start to sweat because you
are nervous, or feeling emotional, or
sometimes just because.

Sweating is an important way that
your body stays cool. Your body likes
to stay around 98.6 degrees Fahren-
heit, or 37 degrees Celsius, and it
has special ways to keep your temperature
just right.

Here's how it works. When you get hot,
your brain sends signals to your body to
start sweating. As sweat evaporates from
your skin, it cools you down because as the
water leaves your skin through evapora-
tion, it takes the extra heat away and you
feel cooler.

Fun Fact: If you could collect
all the sweat you produce, even
in a day, you would be amazed!
In fact, during puberty, a guy that
is well hydrated and exercising
really hard can sweat enough in
one hour to fill 6 soda cans with
pure sweat!

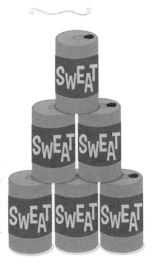

Body Odor

Besides sweating more in puberty, your sweat also takes on
a new smell, especially around your armpits, privates, and feet.
You may not be the first one to notice it, but the people around
you probably will! It's called body odor (or BO), and it can be
powerful in a not-so-good way. Some people say it smells like
onions. Some people say it smells like a skunk. Either way, it's
just stinky.

So why does your sweat start to stink in puberty? It's because your sweat becomes oilier, and the bacteria that live on your skin really think those oils are yummy. As they digest the oils, the mixture of the bacteria and sweat creates new chemicals, like ammonia, salts, sugars, and other smelly stuff. All of that mixed together stinks! On top of that, if you've been eating a lot of garlic or spices, those odors can come out through your sweat, too, providing an extra helping of pee-yew!

Unstinking

So even if you stink, the good news is that body odor is pretty easy to handle. And how do you do that?

Was your first thought deodorant?

Not so fast. There's something else you have to do first.

WASH! With soap. Every day. Yes. Every day.

Once you hit puberty, it's important to wash with soap and water every day—maybe twice a day sometimes. Soap is important for washing away the bacteria and the sticky, oily stuff that sweat leaves behind. You can't just stand under the shower and sing. You actually have to wash your pits and your privates (with soap!), where all those new glands are hard at work. THEN, after you are clean and dry, you can put on your deodorant in your armpits (but not around your privates).

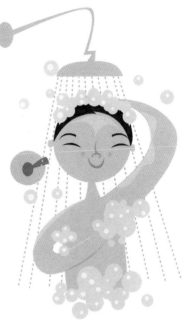

In terms of deodorant, you have plenty of options to choose from. Most deodorant comes with a built-in antiperspirant, too, which helps you sweat less. The deodorant deodorizes you. The antiperspirant stops or decreases the sweat. Most deodorants have a scent or nice smell to them. Deodorants for girls usually smell flowery or fruity. Deodorants for guys usually smell spicy or "sporty." Who made that rule? And how does "sporty" smell, anyway? You can spend a few minutes in the deodorant aisle sniffing and decide which scent you like best, and just in case you can't find a scent you like, there's also unscented (no scent) deodorants.

Unstinking Quickly

If you take a PE class or sometimes even after recess, you may feel like you need to put on more deodorant to keep yourself from smelling. Remember that deodorant doesn't work ON TOP of stink! That means, you have to wipe off the stink, let your pits dry, and THEN you can put more deodorant on. It helps to keep some moist wipes in your locker or backpack for exactly those times.

Fun Fact: Speaking of stink ...do you think you fart more in puberty? No, but the average person farts 14 times a day, and both girls and guys have over 300,000 farts in a lifetime.

Don't think that you can cover the stink with other smells, either. As you are shopping for deodorant or moist wipes, you might see body spray near the deodorant. Body spray is like cologne (perfume for guys). It can help cover smells, but it doesn't stop them! It just puts scent on top of your stink. Most guys and girls learn that too much body spray will keep others away! The best bet is to freshen up with wipes and the deodorant you've come to trust!

The Pits

If you sweat a ton and get big pit stains (wet stains in the armpits of your shirt), you can decrease the sweat better by using your antiperspirant at night after showering (instead of in the morning). If that isn't taking care of the problem, you can try a "clinical strength" deodorant with a higher aluminum chloride level—that's the chemical that decreases the wetness.

The other thing you can do to decrease wet "pit stains" is wear "quick-dry" or other type of noncotton shirts that dry faster than cotton. You can also wear white or black because the pit stains don't show up as well on those colors.

Stinky Feet

What about feet? They get pretty stinky don't they? And yes, your feet sweat, too!

That means that when you shower, you need to wash your feet with soap and water, too. And don't forget between your toes—seriously. **Wash. With Soap. Every day.** Remember?

If your shoes smell, there are a few tricks you can try to decrease the foot funk:

* Don't wear the same shoes all day, every day. They need time to dry out and "freshen up" between wearings (and overnight isn't enough).

* Wear clean cotton socks every day to help absorb the sweat. Don't wear your socks more than once! So in your gym bag each week, pack 5 pairs of socks so you have a

fresh, clean pair every day. Turning them inside out will not work!

* Sprinkle baking soda or body powder in your shoes to help absorb the extra moisture that your socks don't absorb. These powders can also help decrease stinky odors.

* When your shoes are smelly or dirty, wash them in a washing machine to get rid of the bacteria and fungus, then let them dry completely!

* If your feet are sweating and staying in wet shoes too much, you can develop a problem called athlete's foot. This is a fungus (sort of like a mold) that grows around and between toes. It causes redness and itching and sometimes even makes your skin swell, crack, and peel. There are creams, powders, and spray medications for athlete's foot. Most of them are available at your local pharmacy without a prescription. As always, though, see your doctor if the problem is severe or isn't getting better with these simple treatments.

CHAPTER 8

Skin and Hair

Remember the definition of puberty—"to grow hairy or mossy"? Yep, that hair growth starts all over your body once you hit puberty, and you get that visit from the hair ninja. The first place you may notice your hair beginning to grow and get darker is where? Thicker hair on your legs and arms, under

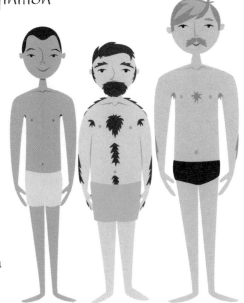

your armpits, in your genital area, and on your face and later on your chest (maybe).

Some men even get hair on their backs!

The appearance of your body hair depends a lot on where your ancestors come from. Everyone has body hair, but on some guys it shows up darker or there's more. For example, if your ancestors are from the Mediterranean region or from Africa, you probably have darker hair. If your ancestors are Scandinavian, it's probably lighter. If your ancestors are from all over, then you might be surprised! That's all there is to it.

For a refresher on how your hair may fill in, you can review the puberty stages in Chapters 3, 4, and 5.

Shaving

So let's talk about those hairy parts. You don't have to do anything for the leg hair or armpit hair. Lucky. Most girls eventually shave those areas (and some guys may shave them for sports or other reasons, but most guys don't—ever!).

Fun Fact: Hair on a guy's face grows faster than hair anywhere else on his body. That's why some men have a "5 o'clock shadow" of hair even though they shaved in the morning

When it's time to shave your face (and that will probably be in late middle school or high school), there are some things to know before you start. You'll definitely need your own razor, and you'll need your parent, an older brother, or someone else to help you learn how to shave carefully and correctly.

Can you just borrow a razor from your parents' bathroom and start shaving? No way! You **never ever ever ever ever ever use anyone else's razor.** Razors can make tiny cuts and pick up blood and skin bacteria that can be passed from one person to another. That can cause skin infections and even pass along dangerous viruses that you don't want.

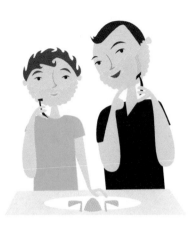

Sometimes, even with a fresh, new razor, you can develop small cuts or red bumps from shaving. If you notice these, make sure you are shaving correctly with a clean razor, a clean face, and using shaving cream. Some guys like to start with an electric razor, which can be a little easier and less dangerous for cuts!

What about using some of Dad's products you may find by his sink, like aftershave or cologne? Be careful. Always ask before using someone else's stuff on your face. The chemicals can be too harsh for your younger skin, or they may cause your face to burn or break out or make you smell a little too strong. Plus, if it belongs to your dad, it's probably best to check with him first.

Skin Care

Along with all of this new body odor and hair comes oily skin for a lot of guys and girls. The oiliness is caused by testosterone, the same hormone that gives you body odor and new hair. What's wrong with oily skin? A little oil is healthy for skin, but

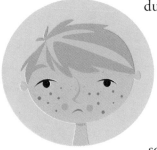

during puberty, there's usually more than your skin needs. The extra oil leads to acne, which means blackheads and pimples, or zits. Zits are the pits!

Most people think of acne as something that happens on the face, but sometimes it shows up on the upper arms, back, and chest, too. Acne seems to be the worst around Puberty Stages 3 to 4, and then it usually starts to get better. **It can be really frustrating and embarrassing to have oily skin and acne, but even the cleanest skin can have it.** A lot of that goes back to your ancestors again. If your parents had bad acne, you may have bad acne, too.

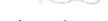

Fun Fact: About 80% of all people between the ages of 8 and 30 have occasional acne break outs.

Acne Dos and Don'ts

If you get pimples, there are some things you can do to help, and there are some things you can do that will make it even worse!

Here's the list of things you SHOULD NOT DO:

- �֎ **Picking.** Don't pick! In fact, picking, pinching, and popping your pimples can cause them to become bigger, take longer to heal, or form scars. So no PPPP (pimple pinching, popping, or picking)!

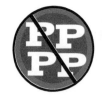

* **Scrubbing.** Scrubbing too hard with a rough cloth or gritty soaps can be harsh on the skin and make acne worse by irritating pores.

* **Covering.** Some guys try to borrow makeup or cover-ups from their mom or a sister. Makeup may clog pores even more and make acne worse. If you want to use a cover-up, make sure it is labeled as "noncomedogenic" (or has the words "won't clog pores" somewhere on the label).

* **Touching.** Touching your face with your hands spreads more oils and bacteria, which can make acne worse. Other things touching your face can be a problem, too. Certain equipment, like helmets or chinstraps, can rub the skin and block pores. If you are wearing equipment that rubs your face, make sure to wash your face with soap and water afterward.

* **Stressing.** Times of stress (like exams, lots of worries, or not getting enough sleep) can make things worse on your face, back, and chest. Stressful times mean more hormones are being released in your body, and some of those hormones can make acne worse. Finding healthy ways to get rid of your stress can help.

Here's the list of things you SHOULD DO to make acne better:

* **Washing.** Washing your face twice a day with a mild soap (or acne soap) and warm water will do the trick for many

guys. Remember not to scrub too hard with rough cloths. Your hands or a soft washcloth are best.

✳ **Eating right.** Eating a balanced diet is good for your skin. That means getting plenty of fruits and vegetables and avoiding too many sugary or greasy foods. Believe it or not, chocolate, sweets, and French fries don't really make acne worse; they just aren't healthy for you.

✳ **Exercising.** Regular exercise will increase the blood flow to your zitty areas, and that helps take away the bacteria and germs that make acne worse. Just remember that after exercising, you need to wash the sweat and dirt off your face and other areas that get zits.

✳ **Removing products.** Try to keep hair products, like gel, mousse, oils, or spray, off your face and hairline. These products can be oily, and they can also block pores.

✳ **Drinking water.** Drinking plenty of water helps keep the skin clear by improving blood circulation and clearing away the bacteria and germs.

If these simple steps aren't controlling your acne and it bothers you, talk with your parents to see if you can use some stronger products from the pharmacy or your doctor. There are a lot of acne soaps, creams, and gels available at the pharmacy. Get a parent to help you choose a mild product with benzoyl peroxide or salicylic acid (those are big words, but they are the

FACE WASH

CLEAN

main ingredients in acne treatments). Both of these can help dry up your skin and make acne better. If you start too strong, your skin will turn red and peel, so read the labels and look at the ingredients.

Whatever steps you take, be patient. **It takes about 6 weeks before you'll see the results of a new product or skin care treatment.** That means you have to do it every day for 6 weeks! If that still doesn't do the trick, you may need to see your doctor. There are lots of other treatments that she or he can recommend to help you.

Acne can be embarrassing and really frustrating. There may be times when you feel like your acne is so bad that no one wants to hang out with you or that you may not even want to go to school. If you ever feel like this, you are not alone. What's important is to let someone (your parent, a counselor, or your doctor) KNOW that you feel like this so you can get help. There are plenty of ways to make it better and help you to feel better about yourself.

Daily Routines Become ... Routine

Taking care of your changing body takes some time to figure out. You may need to experiment with different products, different tricks, and different routines before you find what works best for you and your body. Be patient, and don't be afraid to ask for help if what you're doing isn't working.

MORNING CHECK-LIST

- ☑ BRUSH TEETH
- ☑ WASH FACE
- ☑ GET DRESSED
- ☑ DEODORANT
- ☑ STYLE HAIR
- ☑ MAKE BED

For now, your day may start like this: brush your teeth, wash your face, put on your deodorant, comb your hair. As you get older, you may need to add other steps, such as shaving, taking morning shower, applying acne cream, and maybe even putting gel in your hair.

As you go through puberty, you will find that doing the same daily routine makes it easier to get important stuff done.

CHAPTER 9

Growing Is Hard Work

If puberty is all about "growing" into an adult body, then there's a lot more to it than just testicles and hair, right? There's that part about getting taller and more muscular and not looking like a little boy anymore. That's the part that really starts to amaze the adults in your life. One day you are a little kid, always looking up at the adults around you, and within a year or two, all your pants are too short and you are actually looking eye-to-eye with adults. It's one more amazing thing about puberty.

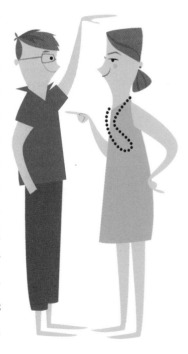

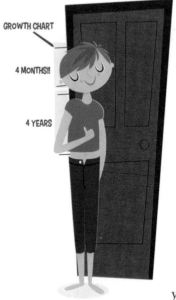

GROWTH CHART

4 MONTHS!!

4 YEARS

It's not like you haven't been growing and suddenly, in puberty, you do. It's just that you've never grown so fast! That's why it can hurt sometimes. (Yes, growing pains are real! For a refresher on normal growing pains, turn back to page 20) Remember that the puberty growth spurt starts with your hands and feet. Then your arms and legs grow. And finally, your trunk gets longer.

In the first part of this book, we told you a lot of what you need to KNOW. Now, let's talk some about what you can DO to help your body stay healthy and feel good while it's growing so much.

Growing

Wow. You are going to get a LOT taller! Think about how many inches guys grow during puberty. You can do that by thinking about the puberty stages:

Normal growth is about 2 inches a year up until you enter Stage 3. Then you take off! Not so fast at first, but you can grow an average of almost 4 inches a year for a few years. So that's usually over a foot; 12 inches that is! Remember that's not exact, but it's an average amount of growth. How much you grow depends on how tall your parents are and how tall your other relatives are. In fact, a lot of doctors use a special math problem (called a

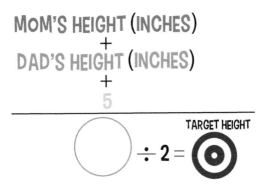

formula) to predict how tall you will be. When you calculate the answer, you'll have your predicted height in inches.

Write that answer down somewhere so you can see if it comes true.

Healthy Matters

It may not seem like it, but growing is hard work for your body. In fact, another thing that affects how you grow is how well you treat your growing body. **To grow in a healthy and normal way, your body needs to be fed well, exercised well, and rested well.** While you are doing all this growing, it is really important to develop healthy habits. Believe it or not, the healthy habits you start now can help you through the rest of your life.

Unhealthy habits (like trying to live on sodas, ice cream, and potato chips or letting your computer keyboard provide your only exercise) are hard to break! Healthy habits can even help you live longer. **So, right now is the perfect time to make a promise to yourself to start eating healthy, getting regular exercise, and getting enough sleep.** That way, all this growing that you're doing will give you a new look that looks and feels great on you!

Here are some simple tips for a healthier you:

* Never skip breakfast! This
  is what wakes your brain
  up every morning. It's like
  starting your engine. You
  just want to make sure your
  breakfast has some protein and
  some healthy energy (carbs). It
  doesn't have to be traditional
  breakfast foods—sometimes
  it's hard to eat a big breakfast
  before school. When you're
  in a hurry, try some of these
  things instead:

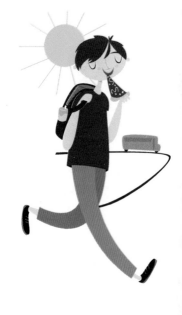

    * peanut butter and jelly
      sandwich

    * leftover pizza

    * a piece of cheese with whole
      wheat toast

Fun Fact: Americans eat about 7 acres of pizza every day! Breakfast pizza may help with that!

    * a smoothie with fruit and yogurt or milk

* What you DON'T want for breakfast is something super
  sugary or that has no protein. A toaster tart or doughnut
  may taste good, but it's not healthy, and it won't last.
  Breakfasts like that just leave you feeling hungry again
  too soon.

✳ Eat small but healthy snacks between meals. Try things like almonds, cheese, an apple with peanut butter, yogurt, or granola.

✳ Don't forget 5 to 6 servings of fruits and veggies every day (the more color on your plate, the better!). Color from fruits and veggies helps provide important vitamins and minerals to help you grow. Try to eat one thing red, one thing orange, and 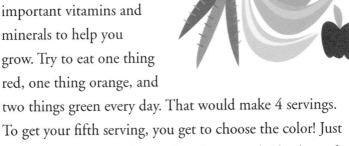 two things green every day. That would make 4 servings. To get your fifth serving, you get to choose the color! Just remember that the color needs to be natural. Skittles and Jell-O don't count!

✳ Let "sweets" be special treats, not a daily habit. That means you shouldn't have dessert with every meal and you shouldn't drink sodas every day. If you save your sweets for special occasions or as a special "treat," it will feel "special" and you'll be healthier.

✳ Eat brown, not white, when it comes to grains, breads, and pastas. Try whole wheat pasta, breads, and even pizza dough. It may take you awhile to get used to the different taste and texture, but getting rid of the white stuff is a big step toward eating healthier.

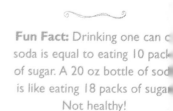

* Drink 6 to 8 glasses of water every day (really!). Water keeps your skin clear, your body healthy, and your brain working better. Your body is made of mostly water, so you need lots of it to keep it "fresh" and healthy.

Fun Fact: Drinking one can c soda is equal to eating 10 pack of sugar. A 20 oz bottle of sod is like eating 18 packs of sugar Not healthy!

* Stay away from soda and any drink that lists any type of "syrup" or "sugar" as one of the first few ingredients on the label. There is a lot of hype these days about sports and energy drinks. The truth is, you don't need any added sugar or electrolytes if you are just playing around with friends in your neighborhood or even having a soccer game that lasts less than an hour. But, if you are sweating a ton and working hard for over an hour, then some of the sport drinks may be good for you. But again, check the label for "sugar" or other fake sugars (such as aspartame, fructose, or corn syrup). If those are on the label, it's not a great sports drink.

* What about the energy drinks? Most of them have caffeine or unhealthy chemicals in them, and you just don't need that at your age. In fact, the high energy drinks can make you feel weird, and they can be dangerous.

* **Exercise for at least one hour every day** (it doesn't have to be all at once). Exercise brings out the best in you. All you need is an hour of active time to keep you running like a well-oiled machine. Try to do things like take the stairs, walk the dog, bike or skateboard when hanging with your friends. Just try to be active in your free time instead of watching TV or playing video games all the time.

* Sleep at least 8 to 9 hours every night Most guys your age should be going to bed before 9:00 on school nights

Fun Fact: You can survive without eating for several weeks. But you can survive only about 11 days with no sleep.

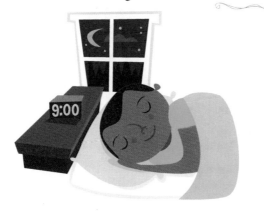

if you have to get up around 6:30 or 7:00 a.m. That would give you the right amount of sleep to keep you healthiest. There are a lot of things happening in your brain and body when you sleep—like storing things in your memory, healing injuries, and growing. That makes it super important to get enough sleep when you're your age. It's also important to realize that **when you don't get enough sleep, it can slow down your thinking and make you grumpy, hungry, and weak.**

Treat It Well!

All this growing and changing can leave you feeling confused, embarrassed, or downright unhappy with the way your body

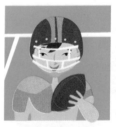
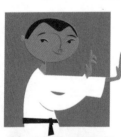
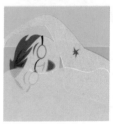
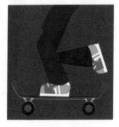

looks. Feel too skinny? Not muscular enough? It can all be very frustrating! What's most important to remember is that your body is changing every day and will continue to change! Most of these changes will help you accomplish amazing things, but you have to continue to take care of your body with healthy eating and drinking, exercise, and rest.

The coolest thing about growing and this time of your life is that you are not a little kid anymore. You are becoming stronger, smarter, and better at complicated stuff. You're gaining a lot of new skills. Look around. There are guys your age that can do backflips, score soccer goals, build robots, write a song, run a 10K race, or do an ollie kickflip on a skateboard. What cool things are you learning to do? If you treat your body well and appreciate all that it can do for you, you may be surprised by how awesome it feels!

Before you know it, you are growing, growing, then grown!

CHAPTER 10

Oh, Boy, Let's Talk About Girls

Now that we got a lot of guy stuff out of the way, let's switch gears here and talk about something different . . . very different.

Girls!

Yep. This is a Guyology book, but we need to spend some time talking about girls, too. Do girls go through puberty? Of course! Just like boy bodies change so they can help with repopulating, girls' bodies change for the same reason.

There are some changes that are similar for boys and girls, but there is also some puberty stuff that is very different for girls than for boys.

72

Why does it matter to you right now? Because **smart guys understand girls**. So let's make sure you understand girls' bodies and the changes that they go through during puberty.

Breasts (aka Boobs)

First of all, girls have breasts. Duh. Boys have breasts, too. But girls' breasts are different, aren't they? Some guys seem pretty interested in girls' breasts. Maybe that's because guys don't have breasts like girls.

By the way, why do girls' breasts need to grow? (Hint: it's not for decoration.) Their breasts grow and develop so that they can make milk to feed a baby. That's pretty amazing: a baby can live off of nothing but breast milk for months!

And just like you probably like to keep your puberty stuff private, so do girls. But when it comes to privacy, it seems that guys have an advantage over girls. As a guy, your first changes are happening inside your pants, where nobody can really tell what's going on. Remember those testes?

The Beginning

For girls, puberty usually starts with their breasts growing. And their breasts are right out in front and noticeable. That makes it tough for girls to hide their puberty happenings. Just like it's awkward when your puberty stuff starts happening, it is awkward for girls, too. And just like you don't want to be teased about puberty, neither do girls. **Teasing about body changes is not cool, and it's not OK.**

The other thing you need to know about girls is that they usually start puberty before boys do. Some girls will start puberty as young as 7 or 8 years old. Others may not start until 11 or 12. That means it's normal for girls to start growing breasts as early as the second or third grade or as late as the sixth grade.

And what about size? Just like guys have penises that are different shapes and sizes (and size doesn't prove anything), girls' breasts come in different shapes and sizes. Bigger always seems to get more attention, but bigger doesn't always mean better. Any size breast can make enough milk to feed a baby.

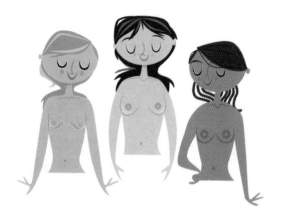

Girls' Private Parts

You have some pretty special names for your guy-parts, don't you? Are there special or funny names for girls' private parts, too? Sure there are. You may or may not have heard some of them, but we're going to go through the correct names.

Remember how we talked about your parts hanging right there in front for you to see and handle? Guys have it pretty easy when it comes to seeing what they've got. Girls' parts are different. Their private parts are hidden between their legs and protected by some folds. That area is called the **vulva**.

Girls have a couple of parts with the same names as yours: the **urethra** (pee hole) and the **anus** (which is not officially part of the vulva). But girls have another opening in the vulva, and it's called the **vagina** (va JIE nah). You've probably heard of it.

The vagina is where a baby comes out when it's born; that's why it's also called the birth canal.

Surprise!

So, now you know: babies do NOT come out of a woman's belly button or her butt. **Babies (and not just human babies, but all mammals) are born through a vagina**. It's pretty amazing how that happens.

And now that you know a baby comes out of a vagina, you should know that babies don't grow in a tummy or a stomach. That would be nasty floating around with all that chewed up food. **Babies actually grow in something called a uterus**. A uterus is an inside part of a woman that is connected to the vagina. So

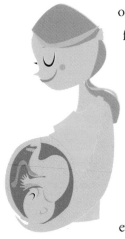

once that baby is ready to be born, there's a perfect way for it to get out.

Sometimes, for various reasons, a baby can't get out through the vagina, so it is delivered by C-section. A C-section is when a doctor uses a scalpel (a really sharp surgical knife) to cut through a woman's lower abdomen and into the uterus, then delivers the baby out through the opening. In the United States, about one out of every three or four babies is delivered by C-section, but most are delivered through the vagina.

Do you have a vagina or a uterus? Nope. You don't need them since men don't have babies!

Other Puberty Stuff

Along with their breasts growing, girls are going through some of the same stuff that you'll go through. Their legs get hairier, they get pubic hair and underarm hair, and they get body odor and acne. And they start growing pretty fast, too.

But there's another part of puberty for girls that boys DON'T go through. Girls get something called a period.

Periods

Have you heard the word "period" before? Well, sure. It's the dot that marks the end of a sentence. But there's another type of period, and it's part of girls' puberty.

When a girl starts having her period, she has some bloody fluid that comes from her vagina for a few days each month. It sounds scary, but it's totally normal, and it's supposed to happen. Most girls start having periods around age 12, but some may start as young as 9 or as old as 16. Periods stop when a woman is around 50 years old. A period is also called a menstrual cycle, or menstruation.

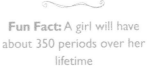

Fun Fact: A girl will have about 350 periods over her lifetime

We're telling you this because it's important for you to know that just like erections can be embarrassing or bothersome for guys, periods can be embarrassing or bothersome for girls. So girls and guys both have strange new stuff going on, and it's important to be respectful of each other. These changes may take a little while to get used to, but soon enough, they seem like no big deal.

Pads and Tampons

When a girl has her period, she will wear a special pad or tampon to absorb the bloody fluid (also called her menstrual flow) so it doesn't get on her underwear and clothes. A pad sticks in her underwear and catches the flow that comes out of the vagina. A tampon is a very small pad-like thing that slips into the vagina to absorb the period flow before it comes out. Tampons have a string on them so they can be taken out easily. Here are some pictures just so you will know what these look like.

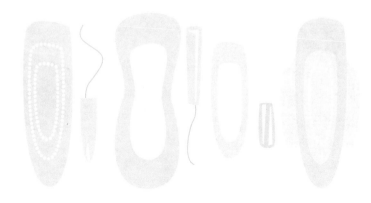

You may see these in a girl's purse, backpack, or locker. Again, it's nothing to tease about—just part of life for a girl. And, by the way, if you do tease her, she'll think you're totally immature. Don't even go there.

Do you have a sister? How about a mother? **Think about the girls and women in your life before you start teasing or picking on a girl about her body.** She's somebody's daughter or sister, too.

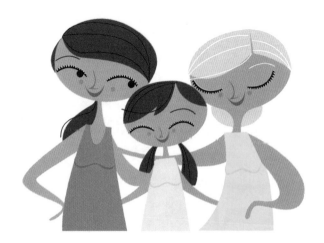

Curiosity

One thing we know about boys your age is that they are a pretty curious bunch. As you start puberty and see other girls and guys having body changes, it's normal to be curious. You may wonder if your body is changing like other guys'. You may wonder about changing bodies and mature bodies, and maybe even naked bodies. Women's and girls' breasts become more interesting, too. And it's easy to see them—just walk past Victoria's Secret, right? You may not want people seeing you look, but it's normal to look (and kind of hard not to!).

But what about looking for naked pictures in other places?

You might see some pictures in books or magazines. Sometimes movies have naked people, but those movies are for adults only. So, what about the Internet? You can find anything there, can't you? But wait! Let's talk about this Internet thing for a moment.

The Internet

The most important thing you need to remember about the Internet is that there are no rules about what can be put on it. That means, **nobody checks to see if everything on the Internet is true**. Nobody checks to see if things are appropriate for children. Nobody removes the stuff that is not appropriate. People can put anything on the Internet, and there are no police or rules that keep it safe. That is why many parents and schools have their own rules about how, when, and where you use the Internet.

When there are no rules, what happens? What if there were no rules in a soccer game? Or football? People would misbehave and get hurt. It would create a lot of problems. Well, **on the Internet, there are no rules, so there are definitely things there that can hurt you, scare you, and be very wrong.**

In particular, there is bad stuff called **pornography** (or porn) that some very wrong people put on the Internet. Pornography is not just wrong and inaccurate, it's dangerous. It involves photos or videos of naked people (actually actors) doing stuff that is very different from what normal people do. It often shows violence and is very disrespectful to women and even to men, too. Most of all, it can mess up your ideas about what's OK and not OK, and it can even scare you.

So, the Internet is no place to look for pictures of naked people. There are too many dangerous places you can land with pictures that you are not prepared to see. Even most adults don't want to see them because they are wrong and just really bad. **And once you see pictures that are wrong or bad, you can't "un-see" them** so they can stay in your mind and bother you for a long time!

What If I See It?

If you spend any time on the Internet, you might land on pornography at some point. It may have already happened to you. Sometimes it just pops up on your screen when you are looking for other stuff. Other times, you may search for something that accidentally takes you there.

If that happens, it's best to close the screen and let a parent know what happened. Don't click on any other buttons on the screen.

What you see may shock or scare you. Most of all, know that if you are seeing porn, it is not the way normal people act. Even the bodies aren't normal, so you aren't seeing anything real. It's all made up to be shocking. By turning it off, you'll keep yourself from having wrong information and from having bad memories of it.

Curiosity Is Normal, But Find Healthy Ways to Get Answers

So, if you are just curious, there are other things you can do. There are safe books you can look through. Your local library has books that your parents can check out. It might be embarrassing to ask a parent if you can see pictures of naked people, but seeing them in a safe book is a lot better then seeing pornography.

Remember, that all bodies come in different sizes, shapes, and even colors. So there is no right or wrong body shape—they're all unique.

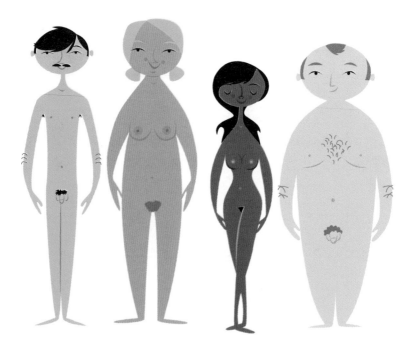

Obviously, you want accurate information. You want to know what's real. You want to know the facts. You want to be right. Your parents are the best way to learn, so if you want to see pictures, you need to ask a parent to guide you so you can get good information that is safe and correct.

What About Real-Life Nakedness?

Every family is different when it comes to being naked. Some parents don't close the door when they are getting dressed. Some families share a bathroom and see each other getting in and out of the shower. Other families encourage closed doors and privacy when it comes to naked times. Within your family, seeing naked bodies can be normal.

Outside of families, though, you shouldn't be seeing other naked bodies or showing off yours. If you have to change clothes in a locker room with other guys, that's different. It becomes a problem when you go out of your way to see other people naked. If you feel like you need to put pressure on younger kids or talk them into letting you see or touch their private parts, that's a problem, too. This is another type of sexual abuse, and it's wrong.

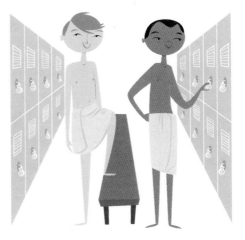

If you become so curious that you find yourself trying to see or touch naked bodies of friends or younger children, you should talk to a parent or your doctor. **Besides being illegal, sexual abuse is harmful in a lot of ways.** The good news is that there are ways to help people stop doing that, but the longer it goes on, the harder it is to stop. If you ever find yourself in that situation or know of a friend who's involved, it's super important to talk to an adult so you can get help for yourself or the other person. That's how we stop sexual abuse.

CHAPTER 11

Feelings and Friends

Obviously, there's a lot of growing going on in puberty. We've mentioned all the body changes, but we haven't talked about your brain. Do you realize that your brain is growing and changing like crazy, too? Around the same time you start noticing your body changes, your brain has also kicked into big-time morphs. And it's cool, because your brain is actually growing smarter, faster, and getting ready to learn totally new things. It's also expanding the area that deals with your emotions.

Fun Fact: Your brain is also known as your gray matter. And your gray matter matters! Although it weighs only 3 pounds and 80% of it is made of water, it uses 1/5th of all the oxygen you breathe and has the storage capacity of over 4 terabytes (that's about 4,050 gigabytes!).

Moods and Attitudes

You've probably heard of emotions. Emotions describe the way you are feeling, and they definitely affect your moods. Your feelings, moods, and emotions are actually a really big part of puberty. Part of the reason they become such a big deal is that

your emotions start to feel bigger than ever and they come and go faster than ever. Sometimes that makes adults think you have an "attitude." Sound familiar?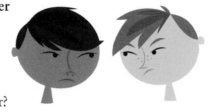

So understanding a little about emotions can help you.

Let's think about all of the different emotions people experience. Go ahead and write down as many emotions as you can think of here:

If you think about all the different types of emotions that people can have, you'll probably notice that some of them are "positive" emotions (like happy, proud, excited, goofy) and some emotions are "negative" (like sad, angry, jealous, frustrated).

Did you notice we said positive and negative but NOT good and bad? That's because **there are no bad emotions**. All emotions are important.

We have to feel happy sometimes. We have to feel angry sometimes. That's normal. But sometimes, people make us feel like we shouldn't show our "negative" emotions, so we try to hide them or keep others from seeing them.

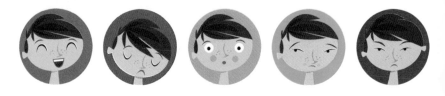

Sometimes we feel comfortable showing our negative feelings only to our parents or our closest friends. When you're with a group of friends, is it hard to cry if you're sad? What about when you're with your family? Maybe it's a little easier.

Negative emotions are a part of life. If you never felt angry or sad, you wouldn't be human. But it's important to realize that the negative emotions should not be the most common (or only!) emotions you feel.

If you find that you are feeling sad, angry, or frustrated most of the time, it is important to find someone to talk to. An adult that is a good listener, like a counselor or a family member, is usually best and most helpful, but sometimes a good friend can help, too. If it's a problem most of the time for you, then it's important to talk with your doctor.

Cool Your Jets

Since it's normal to have negative emotions sometimes, it's super important to learn how to handle them in a healthy way.

How do you "cool down" when you are really angry? Sometimes you may get so angry, you want to break something or hurt someone, but you probably know that those are never the right choices. Instead, think of some things you can do when you are angry so that nobody gets hurt and nothing gets broken.

Here are some ideas:

* Walk away.
* Take 10 slow, deep breaths.
* Do something physical, like running, throwing a ball, hitting a punching bag, doing push-ups until you can't do anymore, shooting hoops, or playing tennis against a wall.
* Talk it out with someone who is a good listener.
* Put on headphones and listen to music.
* Write down what's bugging you, then tear it up.
* Scream into a pillow (but not at a person), punch the pillow (but not a person), flop on your bed, or stomp the floor, but slamming doors and damaging property is not a good idea!
* Play a musical instrument.

It's never good to destroy property or get physical, even if someone else tries to start it first. **And the sooner you learn to control your anger and let it cool down in a healthy way, the more you will be respected and treated like a mature young man**. It takes time and practice to figure out what works best for you, but it's important.

Let Me See You Smile

On the other hand, your positive emotions are easier to manage. People love seeing other people happy. Have you ever noticed that when you're happy or smiling or laughing, your friends want to join you?

Often, your happiness is because you did something awesome, like scored a goal, did well on a test, or got recognized for something you did. Those things will make you proud or excited or just pumped up (those are all emotions)!

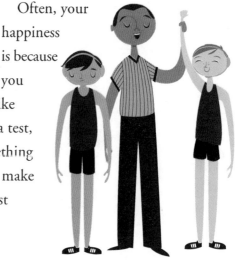

Although you have every right to be happy and enjoy your victory, you may want to make sure your happiness isn't making someone else's sadness or frustration even worse. That's part of being a good sport but not just on the field.

The important thing about showing your happiness is to let it shine, but do it without bragging or boasting. A fist pump and big smile is one thing, but a victory dance that includes poking the "losers" is nothing but annoying and rude. If you must do a victory dance, save it for when you are in a place where you won't annoy or be rude to others who may not be as happy as you are.

Being sensitive to the way other people are feeling is just one more part of learning how to deal with your own emotions and express them in healthy and respectful ways.

Friendships and Relationships

It's impossible to figure out all this emotion and feelings stuff quickly. It takes time and practice, but if you pay attention, you will learn a lot. And you'll find that whether you are cranky, excited, angry, or just somewhere in the middle, it will also affect your friends and friendships.

Most guys don't spend a lot of time thinking about their buddies' feelings. But when you learn to manage your own feelings, you'll realize that feeling angry or frustrated or embarrassed is no fun. And you'll also realize that making other people feel those negative emotions isn't really fun, either. **It feels a lot better to make others smile and feel great!**

Sometimes that's hard to learn. But if you are paying attention, you'll see that making others feel small (sad, jealous, angry, frustrated) doesn't make you feel better. So, you just need to be the guy that doesn't need to feel big by making other guys feel small. That's weak. Got it?

Feeling Shrimpy?

The other thing that affects guys' feelings a lot is body stuff. Changing bodies, and more commonly, bodies that HAVEN'T changed, are often a source of teasing for guys. Sometimes if you feel smaller than everyone else, it can make you want to hide, so you slump your shoulders and look

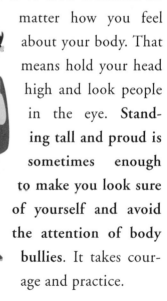

down because you're just not feeling confident. The best way to avoid getting teased is to look confident no matter how you feel about your body. That means hold your head high and look people in the eye. **Standing tall and proud is sometimes enough to make you look sure of yourself and avoid the attention of body bullies.** It takes courage and practice.

What if you're bigger than your friends? Does that mean you can tease them? Both girls and guys get teased about body issues, and does it help anything? Not a bit.

Does it feel good to make someone else feel bad?

Does it make you look cool?

No. It really makes you look like a jerk.

So how should we treat other people?

Have you ever heard of the Golden Rule? It says to **treat other people the way you want to be treated.** If you do that, you'll be doing a great job.

It also helps to think about being a good sport—that means you respect your teammates and you work together to win. Think of all the guys around you as being on one big team, trying to get through puberty. It's a tough game, but if you support each other and don't put each other down, you'll all come out winners.

Girl Friends

Now, what about your friends that are girls? Girls have feelings, too. And during puberty, their emotions and your emotions can get confusing.

Some of your girl friends will stay just that—great friends—but sometimes guys with girl friends get teased about having a "girlfriend."

When do girl friends become "girlfriends"? That's hard to say, but some of the girls around you may make you feel different—like you're not sure how to act around them anymore.

Do you get sweaty palms around them? Do you do something weird or annoying to get their attention? Or maybe you can't talk around certain girls anymore. Puberty, brain changes, and hormones make guys act differently around girls. And they definitely make girls act differently around guys. Maybe there's a girl doing weird or annoying things to get your attention. Part of the reason girls and guys start acting differently may be because of these changing feelings. At some point in puberty, most girls and guys see each other as more cute and less gross.

> **Fun Fact:** On average, a woman speaks about 7,000 words a day. A man speaks about 2,000 a day.

Sometimes, your friends or girls you know may be pressuring you to "like" a certain girl when you really don't have any special feelings for girls at all. Sometimes those special feelings don't happen until later, like when you're a teenager. That's normal, so there's nothing wrong with you if you don't "like" girls. And for some guys those special feelings never happen around girls.

So, this whole "girlfriend" thing can be confusing and frustrating, but there's plenty of time to figure it out. Be patient with yourself, be patient with the girls, and don't pressure your friends. If you think you have a crush on someone, the best way to get noticed is to just be your normal, nice self. Doing goofy and annoying things will get attention, but it's not the kind of attention you want from a crush. And if you don't have a crush? No worries. One day it might happen, but there's no rush.

Growing Up

Learning to be a good friend and finding good friends are only a couple of the prizes that come with growing up. Growing up also means having more freedom, getting really good at the things you like to do, being able to do more things by yourself or with your friends, and getting smarter and smarter. Oh, and of course, growing up also means "growing" into your new body and feelings with confidence, pride, and a promise to take good care of yourself.

The End and the Beginning

Although you've reached the end of this book, it may be just the beginning of puberty. You'll be doing a lot of growing up for years to come. But now that you've learned about all the things that will happen, you don't have to wonder or worry if you're ever going to look older. You know you will. **You'll grow your own unique and awesome look on your own time schedule.**

Reading a book like this also helps you realize that the word "puberty" doesn't need to make you feel awkward. That's because you know it's not just about pubic hair and voice cracks, but it's about bigger and more important stuff than that.

So, yes, you will get a more manly "look," but you will also become more mature. You'll have new skills, new smarts, and new feelings, too. Those are the things that will help you build your confidence and turn you into the respected guy that you want to be.

We hope that this book has given you a lot of the information you'll need. However, if you're like all the other guys we talk with, **we know you'll need more information as you get older.** Getting accurate information is super important, especially when it comes to things like puberty, girls, and growing up.

To make sure you get the facts, it's always best to go to a parent or trusted adult. The person that gave you this book is probably a great place to start. It may feel awkward to talk about things, but the good news is that all adults have survived puberty and they have some great information to help! They know more than you would ever imagine! And if they seem unsure or confused, point them toward Guyology, and we'll keep helping!

Acknowledgements

After a decade of focusing on girl's health and development, it was very refreshing to spend some focused time on boys. This was particularly fun because we were able to involve a group of physicians who care for adolescent boys, the parents of boys who have been nudging us to write this book, and most of all, a great group of teen and young adult guys who gave us honest and often hilarious answers to our many awkward questions for them.

A special thanks goes to Dr. Michael Guyton who contacted us a few years ago as a resident in internal medicine and pediatrics with an interest in helping us grow Guyology. As an Adolescent Health expert and our official test pilot for our Guyology programs, Mike had great insight and recommendations. We look forward to lots of Guyology years ahead with him.

We also want to thank several families that graciously agreed to serve as our first readers. We think there are clearly some senior editor capabilities among many of them!

All of them were hand selected to bring a variety of perspectives and experiences, and also because we respect the ways they love, nurture and educate their own sons. So to the Chamber, Gallivan, Goldsmith, Herring, Hibbitts, Holmes, Johnson, Kellet, Psenka, Spinella, and Thomas families - we are grateful for your help! You have graced us with stories, advice, grammatical corrections, and confidence as we deliver this latest baby into the world. And to Dr. Neill Herring and Dr. Mary Frances Croswell, we are grateful for your insight as both parents and medical experts.

Finally, to our own families, especially Michael and Steve, thank you for your endless (did we say endless?) support. We love you, and we are grateful for your love and generosity in encouraging us to follow our passions.

With gratitude,
Melisa & Trish

Made in the USA
Columbia, SC
17 May 2018